What Should I Know about MY TEEN?

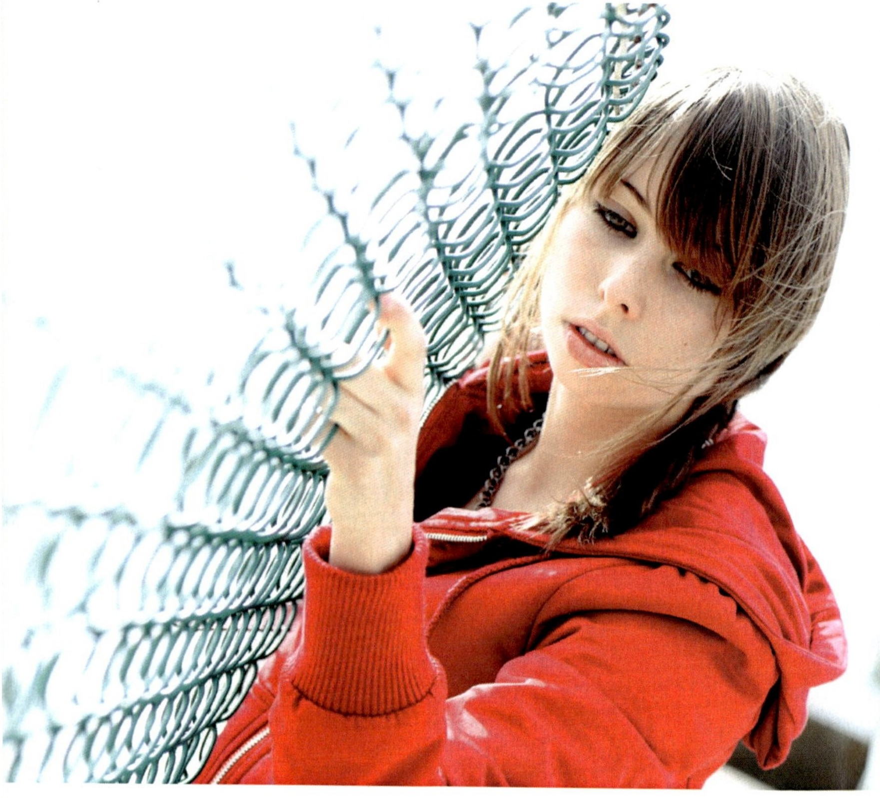

Céline Boisvert

What Should I Know about MY TEEN?

Éditions du
CHU Sainte-Justine

Bibliothèque et Archives nationales du Québec and Library and Archives Canada cataloguing in publication

Boisvert, Céline, 1958-

What should I know about my teen?
(Questions/answers for parents)
Translation of: Que savoir sur mon ado?.
ISBN 978-2-89619-144-4

1. Teenagers - Psychology - Miscellanea. 2. Adolescence - Miscellanea. 3. Parent and teenager - Miscellanea. 4. Teenagers - Mental health - Miscellanea. 5. Teenagers - Sexual behavior - Miscellanea. I. Title.

BF724.B64313 2008 155.5 C2008-942289-9

Cover design : Quatuor
Graphic design: Nicole Tétreault
Cover page photo: Nancy Lessard
Inside photos: Nancy Lessard
Claude Dolbec (pages 8, 25, 33)

Éditions du CHU Sainte-Justine
3175, Côte-Sainte-Catherine
Montreal (Quebec) H3T 1C5
Telephone: (514) 345-4671 • Fax: (514) 345-4631
www.chu-sainte-justine.org/editions

ISBN: 978-2-89619-144-4

Legal Deposit: Bibliothèque et Archives nationales du Québec, 2008
Library and Archives Canada, 2008

The Sainte-Justine Hospital Foundation wishes to thank the generous donors who contributed to *UniverSanté des familles* and made it possible to create this new collection for families.

Thank you for your support... for the love of children!

Table of Contents

About school and the computer

Changing relations

Special means of self-expression

Mental health

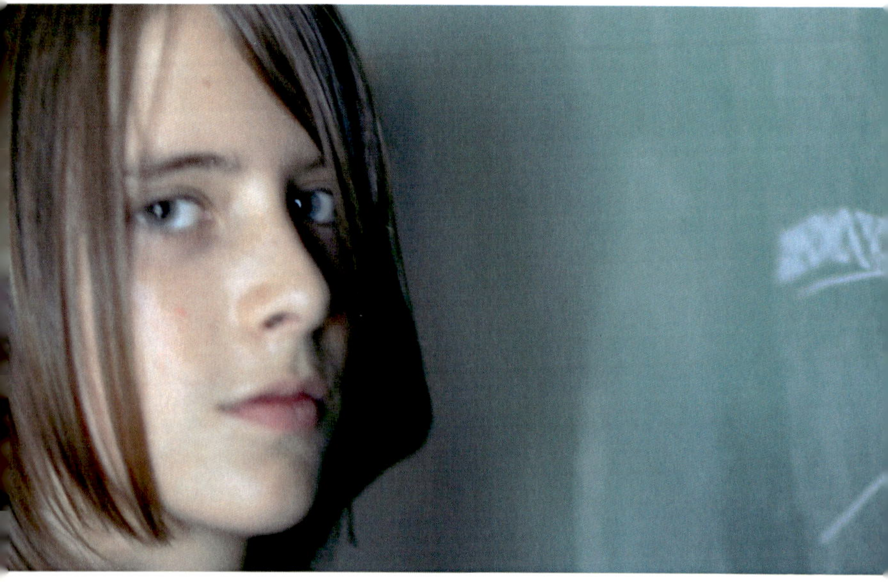

Adolescence identity crisis

What exactly is meant by an "adolescence identity crisis"?

The expression *adolescence identity crisis* has several meanings. It can refer to a passing behavioural disturbance, an inner malaise, conflict with parents, etc. The word *crisis* refers to a sudden, involuntary change in the teen's behaviour, thoughts, relationships and emotions.

We sometimes notice that our teens feel badly about themselves yet are unable to explain why. Their changing moods are an almost unmistakable sign of an inner discomfort they cannot quite put into words. This is caused by internal pressure, of which the teen is more or less aware, that is associated with new and unfamiliar tasks. Because the young person is not actively performing these tasks and has not yet mastered them, they make him nervous. These may be related to the first sexual experience; teens may feel pressured by friends to go ahead and have intercourse. Or they may feel obliged to make quick choices, for example, state opinions on politics, music and other subjects, which can be stressful because these opinions may put them in conflict with parental values, your values, for the first time.

However, rest assured: research has demonstrated that the majority of teenagers do not experience intense or long-lasting conflicts with their parents. Moreover, not all find this time of life difficult and unsettling. With some teens, we notice only subtle shifts of mood and opinion, though even these indicate that important transformations are taking place inside them.

So don't worry too much about the notorious adolescence identity crisis: it is a normal and necessary stage. It will complicate your life and your child's for a limited time only.

Sex-related issues

Don't you think that young people become sexually active far too early? How can we convince our teens to wait until they are more mature?

You are probably right in thinking that today's youth embark on the adventure of sex too early to appreciate its full value. However, when teens decide to have sex for the first time, parents rarely succeed in dissuading them – and then only when they've been previously informed about their child's intentions!

Obviously, nothing is stopping you from giving your opinion, but the teen's decision of whether or not to have intercourse seems primarily determined by the sex education received and the emotional environment in which it was given. Instead of listing all the things that are forbidden, you'd be better to discuss the importance of mutual respect between partners – and don't be afraid to repeat your advice about contraception and protection against sexually transmitted diseases (STD's).

Recent studies show that the majority of young people who claim to be well-informed about sex continue to hold certain false beliefs, for example, that it is impossible for a girl to get pregnant the first time she has intercourse. In fact, the majority of teenage pregnancies are the result of their "first time". Moreover, many young people today continue to believe that AIDS is a curable disease. It is up to parents to dispel this idyllic vision of risk-free sex and remind teens of the death threat, alas all too real, that AIDS represents to this day.

We also have to remember that teens frequently let a period of time pass after having sex for the first time. This is particularly true of girls. It's as if this first experience relieves them from certain pressures. Having taken the big step, they feel they measure up to their peers. Some feel they have become adults as a result. They are not necessarily in a hurry to repeat the experience. We may also emphasize that even today, for many young women the main reason for agreeing to having intercourse is so they won't lose their boyfriend.

Did you know?

The teenager is in a some sense a twentieth century "invention". It was only at the end of the nineteenth century that youth (that is, young people) became a fashionable theme, in other words, that the public became interested in the lives and feelings of individuals who were no longer children but not yet adults. Only at the end of WW I did the word teenager come into use to designate people between the ages of twelve and twenty.

It is also possible that your teen will experience something wonderful when having sex for the first time, even if it did happen too soon for your liking. If this is the case, there's no point in stamping the experience with a seal of disapproval and making the teen feel guilty. Instead, continue to encourage your son or daughter to be careful when it comes to sexual protection, and reiterate the fact that sexual relations must occur in an atmosphere of mutual respect.

Should we take it for granted that because our teenagers take sex education at school, they know what comprises adequate sexual protection?

Methods of contraception and sexual protection are generally familiar to teenagers. However, they still don't use them very often. The principal reasons for this are:

- immaturity;
- magical thinking, which makes them believe themselves immune to risks and dangers, for a variety of reasons;
- they go along with what they are told by their partner of the moment, who encourages them not to use protection;
- they don't dare refuse unprotected sex for fear of offending the other person;
- they don't want to appear as if they are afraid.

In fact, teenage impulsiveness and love of risk are often the source of irresponsible behaviour as far as sexual protection is concerned, in spite of the information young people are given at school.

Some teens continue to believe that their general level of hygiene protects them from everything. Others harbour all sorts of false convictions, for example, that only homosexuals, drug addicts and recipients of blood transfusions are in danger of contracting AIDS. Quite simply, almost none of them think of AIDS as a deadly disease of a more or less long duration. In their minds, tritherapy, which they have vaguely heard about, provides a cure for this terrible illness. They also forget that sexually-transmitted diseases (STD's) can be difficult to treat, come back repeatedly and even, in some cases (as with chlamydia), leave them sterile.

How can adults help teenagers deal with sexual matters?

The challenge faced by adults advising teens about sex is how to give them the facts without frightening them. Teenagers must not end up associating sex with unpleasantness, irresponsibility, illness and death. All this contradicts the view of sex as a natural and spontaneous urge that brings together two people who love each other in sexual union. Indeed, sex *should* be about pleasure, self-expression, health and life, but today's teenagers face a whole other reality, one our generation did not have to deal with. Today's young people, given the choice, would certainly have preferred things to be otherwise!

Did you know?

Sexual activity starts around 15 years old.

Teenagers need your explanations to be accompanied by positive comments and concrete examples. These might include a brochure illustrating condoms, a diaphragm, birth-control pills, or a pregnancy test with instructions.

▸ What can parents do to protect their teen from becoming pregnant?

As far as the prevention of pregnancy is concerned, parents can do two things.

The first consists of giving the teenager adequate information about situations where she might be at risk. Some social situations can very easily lead to sexual closeness that is not planned or even desired. Take for example a gathering of friends where the teenager is tempted to drink alcohol or smoke some illicit weed, out of pleasure, curiosity, or simply the desire to do what others are doing. The teen becomes more relaxed, less inhibited and thus more vulnerable to boys' advances. Another example: the girl is invited to sleep over at a friend's, and without her knowledge boys have also been invited. As physical closeness between the sexes is always a possibility on these nights away from home, when teens sometimes sleep next to each other in the same room, your daughter could find herself lying next to a boy who may be feeling the pressure of his sex drive more than he would like to. You probably had similar experiences as a teen, the kind of experience one is not really prepared for, and which occurs because at this age we feel the need to do what others are doing.

On such occasions, parents must exercise supervision without being too intrusive – quite a challenge! It goes without saying that teenagers need to know their parents

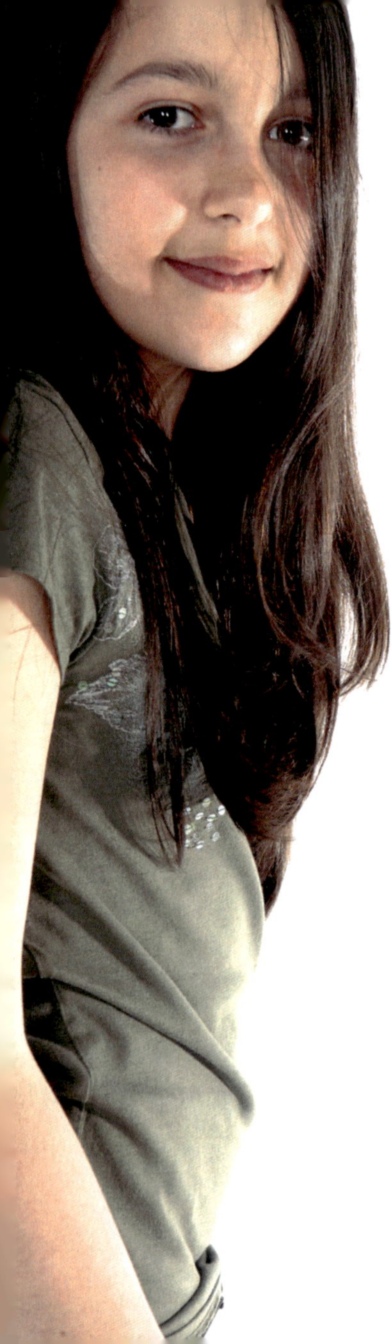

trust them spontaneously, unless they give them reason not to. However, trust does not prevent you from exercising a certain amount of control. Some parents forget that their teens feel the need of a parental presence which by definition creates boundaries. They might not tell you so, but your teens are reassured when you establish limits that are clear without being excessive. For some teens, despite protests, and especially for girls, these limits can even work to their secret advantage. Parental limits mean they don't have to make excuses for refusing to have intercourse. They can explain that their parents won't let them. That way it seems as if it is the parents saying no, not the girl herself. Instead of being laughed at, the young woman will receive sympathy from her friends for having such strict and "backward" parents. And what does it matter if your daughter's friends make disparaging comments about you? Your goal is not to win their approval but to sexually protect your daughter.

However, some parents, wanting to show how open-minded and permissive they are, relax their supervision a little too soon. With this passport to freedom, their teens can party without restraint, sometimes with consequences that are anything but joyful.

The second way of helping your teenage daughter from becoming pregnant is to make sure she uses contraception if she is sexually active. She must decide with her doctor which method suits her best. Naturally, if she is willing, you can discuss it with her. You can also offer to accompany her to the doctor's office. If she agrees, ask if she prefers you to stay in the waiting area or come into the examining room with her. She will appreciate this show of tact and will feel like an adult, taking charge of certain aspects of her life... often with your support.

What can you do if your teen becomes pregnant?

First, you have to know that most pregnant teenagers make their own decisions about the outcome of their pregnancies – and that is the way things should be. But this doesn't necessarily mean that they don't need advice. A young woman who is pregnant most often expects her parents to be supportive and emotionally available to guide her in her decision-making. She doesn't want her parents to make the decision for her out of a belief that "they know what's best for her". Moreover, today in Quebec, from the age of 14 a young woman has the legal right to make the decision herself.

If a teenager decides to keep her child, she can be accommodated, with the baby, in a centre for single mothers. In these centres, the young woman can generally continue her education while the baby goes to an on-site daycare. However, some teens still choose to continue living with their parents. That way, they benefit from the

Did you know?

In Quebec, approximately one teenager out of twelve becomes pregnant before the age of 18. That makes about 4,000 teenage pregnancies each year. The highest rate of pregnancies among young women is recorded in the Greater Montreal region.

financial and practical help that a family can provide, though they must be aware that by choosing to keep their baby, they are irremediably changing the future course of their lives. Indeed, they will face weighty responsibilities for which they will undoubtedly require the help of their own parents.

What if the teenager opts abortion?

In Canada and in France, therapeutic abortion has been allowed for over 30 years. Many hospitals and private clinics offer the service. Resources are available – even to minors – to terminate undesired pregnancies of up to ten weeks. Pregnant teenagers are generally given a lot of information and psychological support from the staff at these clinics.

The physiological after-effects of an abortion are not negligible and include abdominal pain, hormonal disturbance etc., not to mention the psychological effects. Even if the young woman feels relieved after the abortion and doesn't regret her decision, the hormonal changes resulting from the termination will have a temporary effect on her mood. She will have to mourn the child that might have been born, and may feel guilty after the procedure.

Let us note that second-trimester abortions are more complicated to obtain because they represent greater risks to the mother's health and require the use of more complex medical equipment. Finally, let us remember that parents are not always aware that their daughter has had an abortion, because she has the legal right to confidentiality from the age of fourteen.

Why do parents who believe themselves open-minded because they know a few homosexuals react hurtfully when they discover that their child is homosexual?

In spite of our society's growing acceptance of homosexuality, it is not uncommon for parents to fear that one of their children might announce that they are "gay". Faced with their child's homosexuality — no matter how understanding they may be of homosexuality in general — all parents feel grief and go through a mourning of their parental hopes and aspirations. Moreover, certain questions are bound to come up.

After parents have interrogated themselves as fathers and mothers, then as men and women, they may speculate about athletic or artistic activities that they might have encouraged their child to do, to develop a boy's virility or a girl's femininity to better advantage. If you are a parent in this situation, you may also be troubled by images of gay sexual practices that you have never been obliged to think about before and may even consider immoral or "deviant". You may be embarrassed or offended by these images for awhile, then start looking for ways to persuade your teen that he or she is making a mistake, such as holding up the examples of siblings who are not homosexual, though they share the same bloodline and upbringing. You will have to face the fact that this child will not reproduce, except through medically assisted procreation (and then only if their application is accepted), thus depriving you of grandchildren from the bloodline you share.

You will tend to worry about the society in which your homosexual son or lesbian daughter will lead their lives. But remember, your worries may be based on your own experience of society's attitude towards homosexuality, not that of your teen's generation. You are undoubtedly right in thinking that your homosexual child will be exposed to more unavoidable suffering than a young heterosexual. But homosexuality is not a matter of choice; it is a sexual and emotional way of being that is part of who a person is, permeating their senses and fantasies.

Did you know?

There exists no medicine or therapy to "cure" homosexuality, because it is not an illness. When psychological help is sought by homosexuals, it does not aim to "treat" their sexual orientation but the difficulties in daily life that arise as a result of it.

It is very difficult to quantify suffering, for example, to objectively determine if it is more painful to conceal one's homosexuality or live it openly. There are heterosexuals who are far more unhappy than their homosexual counterparts. The gay population does not have a monopoly on life's wounds and burdens. But one thing is sure: the more that people accept his or her sexual preference, the better-adjusted your homosexual child will be. That doesn't mean you agree, it simply means that you love the child enough to continue making them welcome, despite a lifestyle quite different from what you had imagined for them… and for yourself.

You will probably need time to get to this point; all parents evolve at their own pace on the road to accepting their child's homosexuality.

About school and the computer

▸ Our teenager just began high school and seems to have lost his motivation. What should we think about this and what can we do to help?

Entering secondary school puts new demands on teenagers and creates new types of stress that may explain a drop in academic performance and motivation for the first few months. All of a sudden they have a different teacher for each subject and more frequent changes of classroom; they go from being "big kids" at their primary school to being "little kids" at the secondary level, and fear intimidation from older teenagers. Some imagine secondary school as a place where mysterious and frightening things happen, in terms of social and sexual behaviour, drug consumption, styles of dress, etc. After the first months, these fears should fade and the academic performance of your young teen should stabilise, according to their ability.

However, if your child remains anxious and stressed about the transition to secondary school, it is important to identify the reasons for these persistent fears. You may consult various school specialists such as the school psychologist, learning assistance teacher, psychoeducator, level supervisor, etc. The teen who finds it difficult to socialize and adapt to this new academic setting may be lacking in self-reliance. In any case, it's important to react without waiting too long, though it is always preferable to give teens time to find their *own* solutions to the problems you've identified together. However, be aware that "playing the ostrich" about your teen's problems at school is unlikely to make them any better!

Motivation specialists generally recommend that parents follow a few basic principles: establish reasonable goals with the teen; in talking about the work that has been done so far, take the most positive view possible and provide constructive comments; acknowledge the difficulty of the situation, give the teen the "right to be wrong" sometimes. Still, teens must be made responsible in relation to school; it is them and not you who must develop the desire to succeed, though this doesn't mean succeeding every time or doing things perfectly. Young people must also be able to trust the school as a place

Did you know?

Psychoanalysts have gone so far as to claim that it is actually a cause for worry if your child does not go through an adolescence identity crisis, with all its tensions and psychological instability... And everyone knows that it's better to go through an adolescence identity crisis at 15 than at 35 or 50!

of knowledge and skills-acquisition, no matter how many unflattering things they have to say about it. Meanwhile, as parents, you must try to create a good image of the school and communicate your confidence in the teaching staff. It is true that not all teachers have a true calling -- not all are driven by the same psycho-pedagogical ardour! However, blaming teachers for teens' failures makes them lose respect for them; this in turn may incite young people to abandon responsibility for their performance at school.

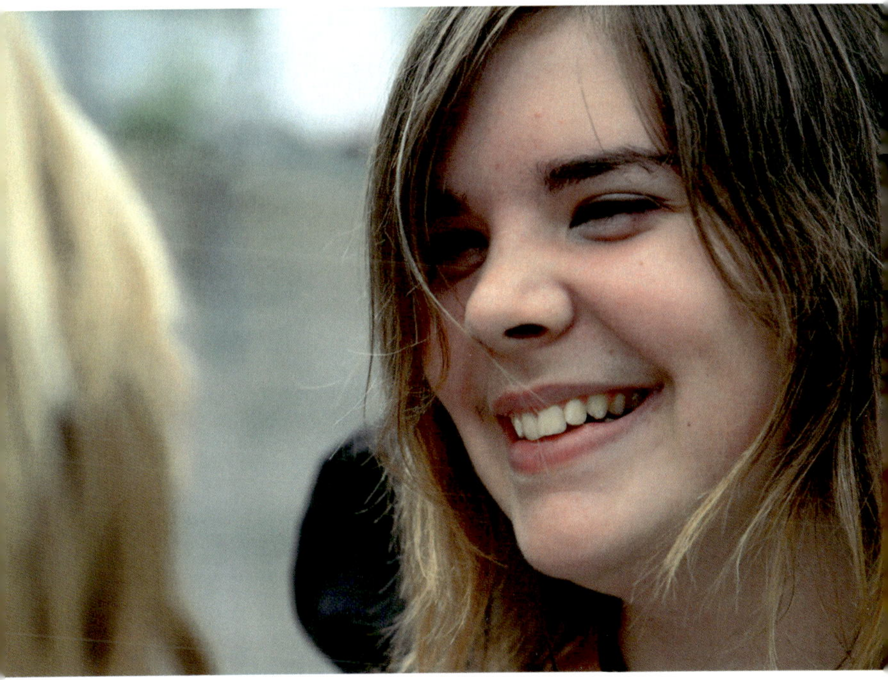

What can we do to prevent our teenager from dropping out of school?

What is the typical profile of a high-school dropout? The candidate is usually a boy from an socio-economically disadvantaged milieu, which generally provides little structure or motivation. This young person has had few positive experiences at school, where he often displays behavioural problems. And if experts have devoted so much energy to drawing the portrait of the high school dropout, it is because the main way of preventing dropout is to identify teens who are at risk.

The signs of a future dropout are as follows: lack of attention to studying and homework, both in class and at home; frequent forgetting of homework to be done, occasional or sustained absences for reasons of physical complaints (nausea, stomach ache, etc.); gradual loss of interest that affects marks and in-class attitude; loss of confidence about the idea of passing and loss of faith in the idea that school is "good for something".

You can help your teens by going over this list of warning signs with them. You may also help them organise schoolwork more efficiently and identify the greatest sources of stress. Offer words of encouragement and

Did you know?

Though statistics vary from one study to another, it is generally estimated that in Quebec, over one teenager in five drops out of school at the secondary level.

establish realistic objectives. You can ask for help from school professionals, who may already have expressed concern about your child's progress in class.

In short, if you feel that your child displays the characteristics of a future dropout, react now! Launch an all-out campaign to shake him up, make him aware, and provide the tools he needs to stay in school. There is far more that can be done before your child drops out than after. Some dropouts "drop back in", but this presents a considerable challenge whose success greatly depends on the young person's temperament and drive. After dropping out, naturally your teen will still welcome your collaboration, but your influence may be limited with young adults of 17, 18 or 19 who will claim to be capable of making their own life choices.

▸ Is it normal for our teenager to spend so much time in front of the computer? What's so interesting about it?

Many parents are concerned and startled by how many hours their children spend in front of the computer. Though they know the computer has become an indispensable tool and realize it is important for their teens to be able to use it, they wonder (quite rightly!) why it occupies so much of their leisure time as well. How does one find the right balance when it comes to internet "chatting", action-packed games and other uses of the computer?

Computer chat

On-line chatting is not in itself harmful or to be discouraged. It promotes exchanges between friends and network contacts. However, two warnings are in order. The **first** concerns random encounters that your child might make on-line. Some dreamy and romantic teenagers, generally young women, get taken in by strangers, in spite of their intelligence and knowledge of the risks.

They may also experience a huge disappointment when they meet their correspondent in person! And disappointment is sometimes the least worrying outcome of these meetings. A chance encounter with a person of questionable intentions can be a traumatic, even dangerous experience. That is why it is important to repeatedly warn your teen, while acknowledging her right to a certain amount of privacy. And if, in spite of knowing the risks, your daughter still wants to meet the person she has been chatting with, make her promise to do so in a public place, discreetly and accompanied at a distance by a friend, an older brother, etc.

A **second** word of caution concerns the fact that these exchanges, though direct, are not quite authentic. The feeling tone that accompanies a message is not always accurately transmitted – or even transmittable. It often happens that a person chatting on-line misreads the other's intentions. Everyone interprets the messages as they can and want to. Distance also creates an illusion of safety and the impression that one can say anything and everything one wishes. The computer helps some people lose their inhibitions and express themselves freely, but this can also create a false impression of who they really are and what they really want to say. If people communicated this way in real life, it would create constant tension and dissatisfaction in a person's relations. Therefore, computer "conversations" must not become your teenager's main way of communicating with others.

Computer games

After spending a few hours at the computer, your teenager will sometimes feel like the ruler of some intergalactic empire or a world race-car champion. Games give him instant gratification. He does not have to work for very long to become the best, and can give free expression to a whole range of emotions that feel genuine, though they are experienced in a context that is totally artificial. Once the game is finished, the young person clicks the off-switch for the computer, and puts away these emotions until next time. This is certainly not the way things happen in real life!

In other words, these games bring a kind of satisfaction that teens rarely experience in everyday life – at least not so quickly and after so little effort. By playing computer games, young people are also spared feelings of wounded pride, for their defeats remain secret. Everything happens between them and the machine they seek to dominate. They never need to lose face or experience "dishonour" – but nor do they experience what is instructive about defeat.

Your teen also risks becoming "addicted" to strong sensations and easy gratification; they risk never discovering the incomparable pleasure and satisfaction that result from sustained, self-driven effort that leads to success. The danger for certain teens is that they will become thrill seekers, satisfied only by strong sensations that are quickly and easily attained. These desires too often lead to passivity, not to speak of the consumption of substances that instantly produce similar sensations.

If your teens are spending hours in front of the computer for reasons other than school work, and continue to ask for more computer time, it is best to start regulating their use of the computer. Access time should be limited, even if you have to resort to using a timer so they won't forget and go overtime. Regularly explain your reasons for doing so, and try to guide teens towards other activities and pastimes. They should be complimented on their abilities and the challenges they set for themselves, for their efforts, successes and good attitude towards difficulty. Still, nothing will guarantee that they will come around to your point of view. We did not grow up in this virtual world and no doubt underestimate its appeal, as well as its positive aspects.

Changing relations

What can we do if we don't like our teenager's group of friends?

Belonging to a "gang" of friends is a rite of passage for most teenagers, a kind of temporary replacement for family support. The very special kind of support that a group of friends provides is almost indispensable for most teenagers. It helps them become gradually less dependent on their families, find their footing and grow up to be more independent.

If you dislike your teen's group of friends, you must say so. But remember, everything is in the way you say it! If you don't like the group's mentality and would prefer that your child stop seeing them, present your arguments with care. If you don't, your son or daughter may use your attitude as an excuse to see this group of friends even more often. Clearly explain why you are not comfortable with this group. Try to avoid emotional reactions such as tears and anger, remaining firm and resolute. It goes without saying that you cannot choose your children's friends – that would be too easy! When we interfere too much in their personal lives, they hold it against us, sometimes hiding who they are seeing, which means we've made no progress at all. Therefore, when your teen brings home a friend whose style and manners offend you, remember that appearances are often deceiving. Try not to judge at first sight. If you start out with an open-minded attitude, your child may be more inclined to consider your opinion later, if you continue to feel uneasy about his or her friends.

Will our teens automatically reject the values we have taught them and favour those of their group of friends?

Rest assured that teens do not necessarily adopt all the values of their gang of friends. Some hook up with people very different from themselves – more rebellious, more marginal or more outspoken. In some sense these friends give them an outlet for their worries about growing up and having to make their own choices. But deep down, they know they will not follow what their group preaches to an extreme. However, if you are sure or have good reason to believe that members of the group take drugs, you must become twice as vigilant and intervene more firmly. Studies have shown that the risk of drug consumption is much greater if a teenager regularly sees a group of people who use drugs. Become informed about drugs with books and articles on the subject. Consult internet sites, a tactic which will set you apart from more old-fashioned parents and provide you with up-to-the-minute information, the internet being the most common source of documentation on the subject.

Finally, be aware that not all teenagers feel the need to spend their free time with a group of friends. Those of a quieter or more solitary temperament prefer to be alone, or in the company of one or two friends at the most. It is possible that their social needs are fulfilled at school. They are not necessarily suffering from not being part of a group, and so there is little point in worrying about it.

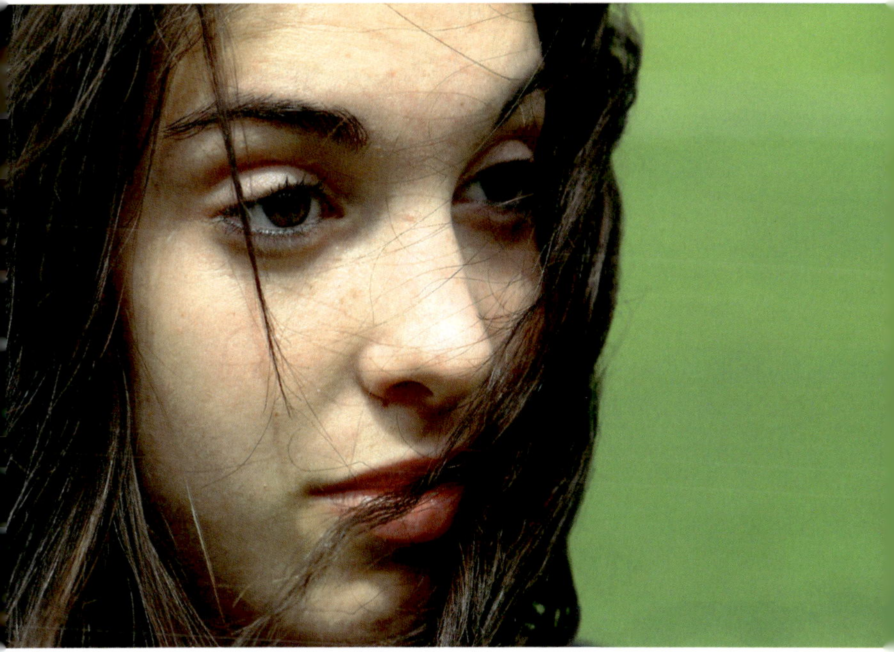

Is it true that teens deal more easily than younger children with parental separation?

Many parents judge that it is preferable to wait until children become teenagers before separating. They feel the separation will be less damaging for teens than for younger children. Indeed, some parents put off their separation until the "baby" of the family has reached the age of 13 or 14.

It is true that teenagers are more capable of logical thought and understanding than young children. For example, they adapt better to moving from one home to another because they are better at orienting themselves in time and space. Still, adolescence being an unsettling time of life in general, some teens will be thrown off balance by parental break-up, sometimes far more than their parents expected.

These teens experience deep sadness that they do not always express for fear of seeming like "big babies". They feel anger, as well as a stress-producing feeling of responsibility for younger siblings, and divided loyalties with regard to their parents. They may also feel guilty and torn about time spent with parents versus time spent with their all-important friends, not to speak of their growing need for freedom.

Like younger children, teens need support, a listening ear and comforting presence, even if they don't demand it as their younger siblings may do. Teens can even seem annoyed by your efforts to encourage them. When deciding on custody arrangements, make sure that teens can maintain contact with their group of friends, an essential source of comfort they will need more than ever.

In case of separation, is it preferable for teenagers to live with one parent rather than the other?

Whether a separation happens before or during adolescence, some thirteen-to-eighteen year olds will feel the need to spend more time with their same-sex parent. This is because it is in some sense more profitable to have that parent around at a time when they are dealing with physical changes and the introduction to sex. It reassures them. It does not have to do with feeling more affection, attachment or love for that parent than for the other. However, some teenagers do not feel this need and prefer to spend equal time with each parent, when possible.

Because of their new social life, teens go out more and get more involved in extracurricular activities. Therefore there must be greater flexibility in the scheduling of time to be spent with each parent. Don't take too strict accounts of the time your teen spends with you. If both the school and group of friends are located in the neighbourhood

Did you know?

Close to 30% of Quebec children and teenagers have parents who are separated? This percentage is even higher in big cities like Montreal. Single parenthood, shared custody, and reconstituted two-parent homes are some examples of the "new family" that work well despite imperfections. But after all, what family can claim to be perfect?

of only one parent, that is where the teen will likely want to stay more often. Show yourself to be adaptable – your teen will be grateful! If you happen to be the parent in whose home the teen is spending more time, you can encourage him or her to spend more time with the other parent. You could suggest, for example, that the other parent could pick the teen up after an evening out or do errands together. If you have experienced major conflicts over the custody of your children, and it is you the teen wants to spend more time with, resist the temptation to gloat about it. To do so will not help your teen at all. To grow up healthy and solid, all children and teenagers need to build positive inner representations of both parents. Being a good parent means being able to recognize and support the child's developmental needs, no matter how stormy the parents' break up may have been. Obviously, at times this will be asking a lot of you.

Special means of self-expression

▸ What are we to think of the tattoo and body-piercing trends that have been adopted by so many young people?

Tattoos and body-piercing are relatively new among teenagers in the Western world, providing them with a special means of self-expression.

Among so-called "primitive" societies, such practices are a way of displaying one's belonging to a group, and can also play a role in special customs; for example, face and body paint is applied for battle or funeral ceremonies.

Today, in the Western world, young people get tattoos and piercings for fun but also to make a personal statement. Unlike their counterparts in certain traditional societies, they do not just want to display their belonging to a group, but to assert their own individuality. The teenager wants to be seen as "different from before". The new mark on the skin or perforation of the flesh signifies – and proves - that he or she is no longer the same.

The majority of young people get just one or two tattoos or body piercings and are just following a fashion. However, others who wish to express something more essential about their developing identity may "overinvest", that is, go overboard, and get tattoos and piercings all over their bodies. This kind of excess can become problematic and slightly distasteful, but it does not necessarily lead to a pathological state. Nonetheless, it is important to be watchful and make sure your teen's "fashion statement" is not turning into a self-harming ritual.

If this does happen, be aware that it is not the fault of tattooing and piercing alone. When teens start harming themselves, for example practising self-mutilation, it is due to a pre-existing disfunction in their relationship to their bodies.

We can forbid teens to acquire tattoos and piercings, limit their number or attempt to dissuade them by quoting the very real risks of infection. What's more, contrary to popular belief, tattoos cannot be removed easily or painlessly, and even when removed, leave behind ugly marks. We can use the example of a game the teen once loved but has ceased to care about. Chances are in a few years, when the fashion has faded and the teen has grown even more, they may not care for their tattoos either.

Can tattooing and body-piercing lead to self-mutilation, a ritual that people say is becoming increasingly common?

Self-mutilation has become increasingly widespread, or at least more incidences have been reported in recent years, especially among teenage girls. However, as we noted above, there is no direct link between tattooing, or piercing, and self-mutilation, though the gestures involved are similar.

Self-mutilation consists of more or less deep scarifications of the skin, generally on the forearms and thighs. In more severe cases, young people seriously injure themselves. One of the dangers of this behaviour is that it is carried out in secret. Teenagers who self-mutilate openly are signalling that something is wrong, or trying to provoke others. Secretive self-mutilation is more pathological, for example, when teenage girls make marks on their bodies and hide them with long, loose clothing. These behaviours are dangerous because they often escalate; there is an increase in the frequency and seriousness of the acts.

Based on the testimonies of teenage girls, we have learned that these acts serve, among other purposes, to relieve stress, inner tension, or the pressure of a problem that they cannot tell anyone. Physical pain, unlike the psychological kind, offers the following "advantage": when a teenager inflicts wounds upon herself, it gives her a sense of control. She controls the experience from beginning to end and this makes her feel she has the power to relieve the tension that she finds so unbearable. Self-mutilation gives her the feeling that she can control her own body and thus, her own problems.

However, for some young woman this behaviour becomes a vicious circle. Through these acts, her tension and deep-seated problems are not solved, but merely displaced. After the few hours or days of relief brought about through self-mutilation, the tension comes back even more strongly. To find new relief, the teen requires an even greater "dose" of self-mutilation.

If you discover that your child is practising self-mutilation, you must contact mental health professionals: psychologists or psychiatrists working in the child psychiatry unit of a hospital or private clinic. If it is not possible to consult these professionals, you can talk to your teenager's general practitioner.

Severe self-mutilation is considered a sign of psychopathology, that is, of mental illness that must be identified and treated. The chances of successful treatment are good, but professional help is absolutely necessary and may end up lasting for quite a long time.

Mental health

▸ They say that teenagers sometimes suffer from anxiety? What exactly does this mean?

An individual suffering from anxiety is overwhelmed by a fear that serious danger lies ahead. The person is tense and experiences various kinds of physical discomfort – acute worry and the feeling he is helpless to prevent the feared events from happening. However, it must be noted that anxiety reactions can also be completely normal, for example, when a teenager has to give a talk in front of the class, perform in an artistic or competitive sports event, ask someone out or be asked out. These are common situations in which most teenagers manage to overcome their stress.

For a state of anxiety to become a source of real suffering, first the teen has to have a neuro-biological predisposition to anxiety, a long-standing nervous, anxious temperament.

▸ What are the most common anxiety disorders among teenagers?

The expression "anxiety disorders" is a general term that includes almost fifteen diagnostic subcategories. The most frequent of these among teenagers are:

- **generalized anxiety**, which means teens have difficulty concentrating in class and elsewhere, are unable to stop thinking obsessively about their problems and whatever else is worrying them. They have trouble sleeping, are tired upon waking; they feel tense and on edge without being able to identify the exact cause of their unease;
- **social phobia and avoidance of school**, a problem that consists of a marked and excessive fear of social or school situations. For example, a teenager finds a thousand-and-one reasons not to have to leave the house, either to go to school or meet with friends. The inability to go to school is becoming a widespread problem, which must be managed on a daily basis and disrupts the life of the entire family. Moreover, under the age of 16 it is illegal to stay out of school, and teens who do so risk failing their year;
- **panic disorder**, when a person experiences repeated attacks of panic that have no precise cause. The onset of attacks is sudden and dramatic, startling the person and everyone around them. Discomfort is intense. The sufferer complains of strange and alarming bodily sensations: palpitations, trembling, muscle spasms, a feeling of suffocation and lack of oxygen. The young person may also perspire profusely, have sharp pains in the chest, stomach, etc., and describe symptoms such as nausea, the fear of fainting, of going insane or even dying.

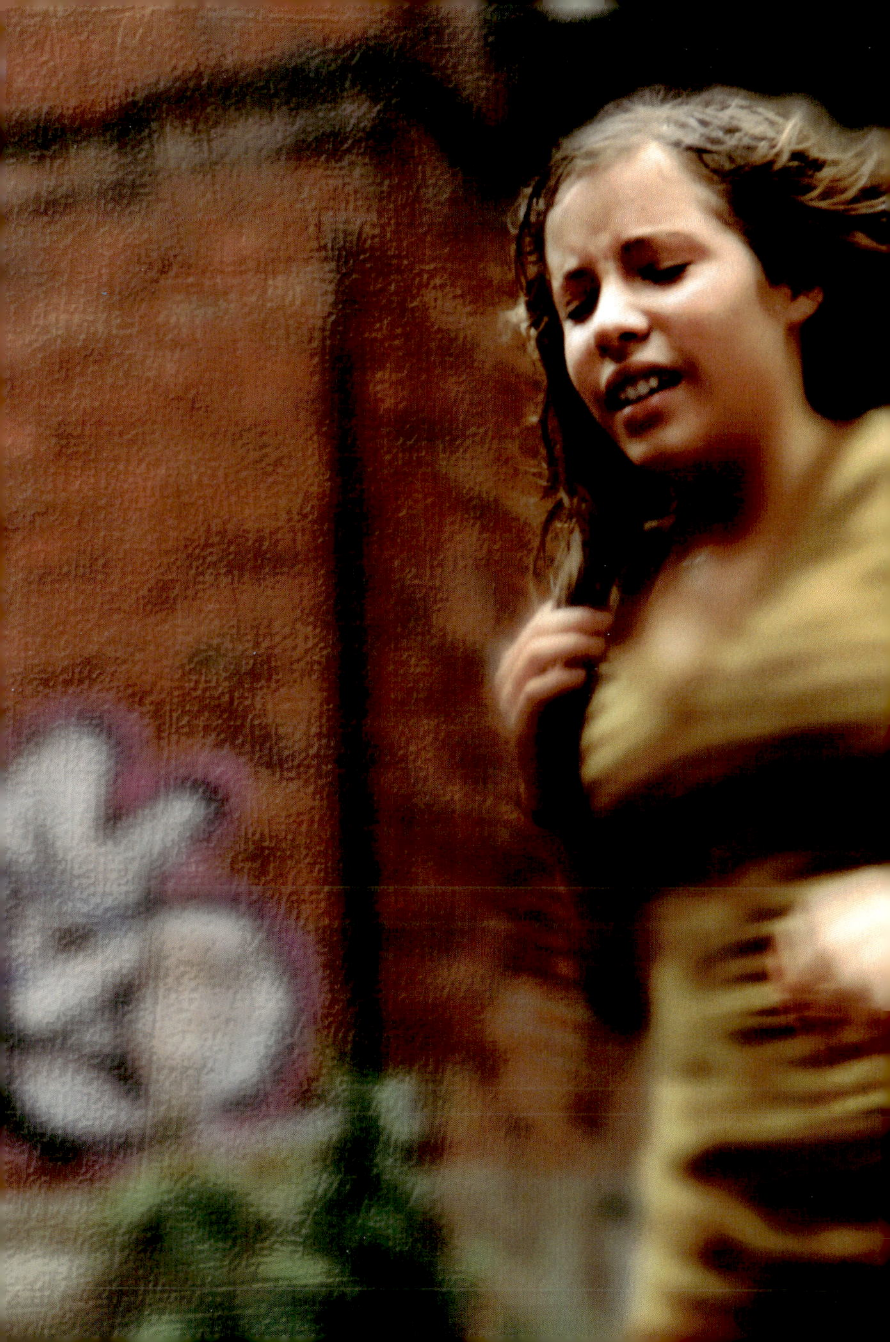

▸ What can we do to help our anxious teenager?

In the three anxiety situations we have just described, teenagers must get help from specialists: psychologists, nurses, social workers, and psychoeducators trained in dealing with anxiety. A general practitioner will usually evaluate the young person and give a referral to a psychologist, at least for part of the treatment (e.g. for psychotherapy sessions). These professionals work either in private practice or in child psychiatry clinics in hospitals.

Serious anxiety can considerably reduce your teen's level of daily functioning. That is why it is advisable to seek help quickly. In the situations described above, psychotherapy is generally recommended. Sessions usually occur once a week at the beginning of treatment, and are gradually spread out.

A person having a panic attack appears physically ill to both himself and the people around him. Therefore, the first step is to see a medical doctor for an evaluation. Generally, these patients are in excellent physical health in spite of all their symptoms. Even if no physical illness is diagnosed, it doesn't mean that the person is not genuinely suffering; the physical pain and discomfort are very real, even though they are of psychological, and not physiological origin. The extreme worry the person feels is quite legitimate and requires treatment, as do any of the physical symptoms.

In the three cases of anxiety previously described, the doctor may prescribe something called an "anxiolytic", that is, a kind of medicine that provides quick temporary relief from extreme states of stress. However, as this medication is not always absolutely necessary, some patients prefer to go without and start directly with psychotherapy. The use of medication depends on the seriousness of the anxiety: if it is acute, the doctor — and often the patient, too — agree that it should be introduced right away. That way, the patient's general state is improved and psychotherapy may be started in parallel.

How can I tell whether my teenager is suffering from depression ?

All teenagers, over the course of their development, will experience normal and variable depressive reactions. These are mild and can occur more than once before disappearing in early adulthood. We must remember that growing up is not easy; teens have mixed feelings about leaving the safety of childhood and facing a future rich with promise but also somewhat frightening.

However, it also happens that the melancholy so typical of young teens does not go away but increases and ends up taking up so much room in their lives that their behaviour is seriously affected. This may be the beginning of depression.

If your teen is becoming depressed, he or she will display five of the signs listed below. These five diagnostic signs or symptoms must be recent developments (that is, you never saw the teen behave this way before) or have got worse (you *have* seen the teen behave this way before, but never to such a degree). These signs must be visible in your teen's behaviour for two weeks without interruption, that is, several times a day, and every day, for two weeks. Your observations can help health professionals to arrive at a diagnosis; moreover, these professionals are the *only* people who can make a diagnosis and determine a course of treatment.

Here, to guide you in your observations, are the signs that may indicate that your teen is becoming depressed.

1) Irritability; frequent bad moods, "grouchiness";
2) sad, depressed mood;
3) loss of interest and pleasure in activities once enjoyed;
4) loss of appetite, pronounced weight loss though the teen is not on a diet, or on the other hand increased appetite and pronounced weight gain;
5) scanty, poor-quality sleep, or on the other hand, sleeping to excess;
6) great restlessness, inability to sit still, or on the other hand great inertia, as compared to the past;
7) constant complaints of fatigue and lack of energy;
8) self-accusations of being useless and incompetent, good-for-nothing, a failure;
9) enormous guilt for no reason;
10) lack of attention and concentration; sharp drop in marks at school;
11) indecisiveness, inability to make choices or take a stand;
12) frequent thoughts of death, even allusions to suicide ("Things would be better for everyone if I were no longer around").

What should we do if our teenager is depressed? What treatment will be prescribed?

If your teenager displays five signs or symptoms from among the twelve listed above, you must consult a health professional.

This could be your family doctor, your child's paediatrician or another doctor, preferably someone who knows the teen a little. The nurse, psychologist or psychoeducational consultant at your child's school can also help you to find a professional to assist you if you don't have a family doctor. If necessary, go to a walk-in clinic or the emergency department at your local hospital.

Did you know?

According to a 1995 study by a Quebec coroner, fewer than 1% of teenagers who had committed suicide had been taking psychotropic medication, that is, medicine used to treat psychiatric problems. Chemical analysis of the young suicide victims' brains showed very low levels of serotonin and its metabolite. The basic molecules contained in many antidepressants are prescribed for this very problem. They aim at raising and restoring the level of serotonin to stabilize moods and help curtail dark thoughts that may provoke suicide attempts.

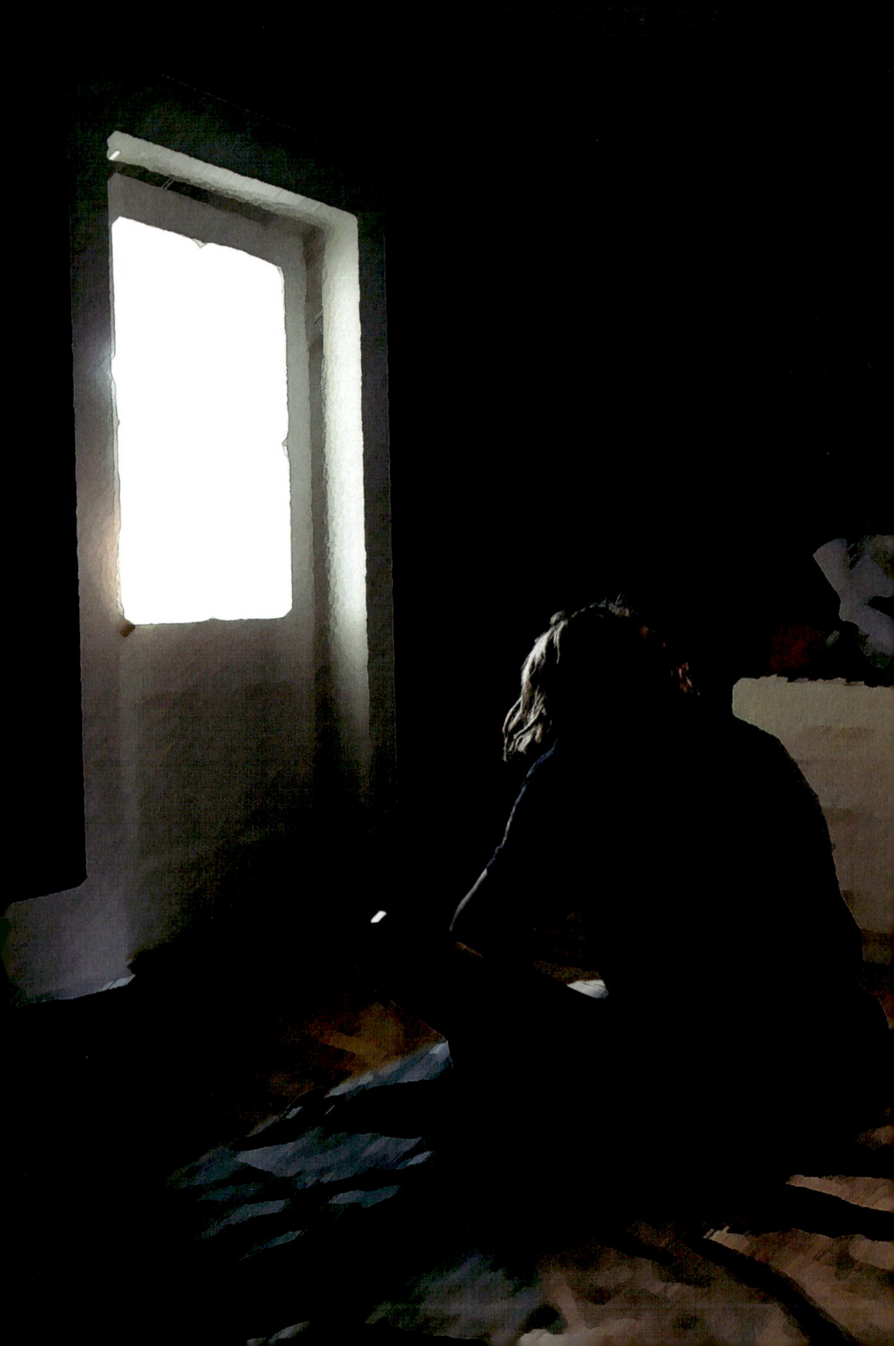

Teenagers diagnosed with depression will be offered treatment. The nature of the treatment will depend on the gravity of the depression, and only the doctor and other health professionals who meet the teen will be able to judge the situation.

Generally, a depressed teenager will be recommended psychotherapy and regular appointments with a specialist who treats young depressed people. At first, these appointments will take place on a weekly basis; when the teen's condition improves, the appointments will be less frequent. In most cases, the young person will also be prescribed an antidepressant to help dispel the most acute symptoms more quickly. Many teens and their parents disagree with the use of medication, and it is their right to refuse it. However, in many cases, medication can prove very helpful. It is essential for you and the prescribing physician to discuss the medication's benefits and side-effects. This kind of medication is generally prescribed for a period of three to twelve months; after that period, the teenager's state will be evaluated and a decision made as to whether the medication will be continued or not.

If your child had pneumonia, you would not hesitate to have him or her take medicine that would cure the illness. It is understandable that you might not feel the same way about medication for mental illnesses, such as depression, because it primarily affects brain functioning. But remember, long studies are conducted before medication is prescribed to young people.

It is important to note that teenagers must have a say in all treatment options. They must *agree* to psychotherapy and medication if you want them to follow the treatment.

How can I tell if my teenager is suicidal?

Teenagers often have depressive moods, moments when they are "down in the dumps" – that is part of their development, and it shouldn't be a great cause for worry.

However, when this period of melancholy and dark thoughts continues, and teens refers to death as a solution to their stress or other problems, if they write or make drawings on the theme of death or listen to music containing references to death, if they start giving away cherished belongings, you must react.

Though it is not pleasant or easy for parents, it is strongly advisable to speak to teens directly about their desire for death and immediately take them to see a professional. In order to get a precise idea of your child's state, it would be useful to get the impressions of close friends who have the opportunity to observe him or her in another context.

What causes a young person to have suicidal thoughts?

It is difficult to identify a single cause for suicidal ideas among young people. They may be anxious or depressed, that is, beginning to suffer from a mental illness, but the cause may also be an outside event. For an emotionally fragile person, this event may act as a "trigger". Teens may become discouraged over bad marks or the falling-through of a cherished project, the break-up of a romance, or any event that upsets their routine, self-confidence and life in general. It is often at such moments, and for reasons having to do with the teen's personality, that death starts to seem like a solution to problems, to humiliation, etc.

Boys are more inclined to react impulsively when they have suicidal ideas. This means that they choose more permanent methods (firearms, hanging), so their rate of suicide is higher than that of girls, who tend more to overdose on medication and are often saved by emergency medical intervention.

▸ What are the main risk factors, that is, the circumstances that most often lead young people to attempt suicide?

- Psychiatric illness – and not only depression – puts a young person in a high-risk category if the illness is not being treated by specialists.
- Drug and alcohol abuse, because these products lower the inhibitions, cloud judgement and often make a person impulsive.
- A combination of the first two factors creates a very high-risk situation.
- Learning that someone close has committed or attempted suicide.
- A "hot-headed" and impulsive temperament in a young person experiencing great difficulties and failures that seriously harm his self-esteem.
- Difficulties with sexual orientation, particularly among boys who discover they are homosexual and live in a milieu that does not tolerate this sexual orientation.
- Easy access to a firearm.
- A previous suicide attempt makes a teenager more likely to try again.

Are there factors that *protect* a person from suicidal thoughts?

Yes. We must keep in mind that alongside the *risk factors* there exist *factors of protection.* These help teens get through difficult and unsettling events in their young lives. The protective factors include family support (in spite of what teens often claim), treatment for a mental health problem, a strong social and friendship network, involvement in projects that keep the young person active, and spiritual values. We must also emphasize that not all teenagers who contemplate suicide on a day of deep discouragement commit this irreparable act.

It is also important to consider that teens who do attempt suicide often get themselves back on track, little by little, using the event as a learning experience that helps them in their future lives. Rest assured that if you do go through this kind of experience with your child, with time and the right professional treatment, hope is often restored.

Did you know?

Between 5% and 7% of children and teenagers suffer from problems with anxiety that are serious enough for them to be given professional treatment?

My daughter is very concerned about her size and often goes on diets to lose weight. Is she developing a problem with anorexia?

Your daughter's dieting will not automatically lead to anorexic behaviour. Watching one's weight is an excellent way of avoiding a number of serious illnesses. But here we are talking about a *healthy* weight; the anorexic's weight is very obviously far below that. The dangerous weight-loss she forces upon herself brings other health problems: a slowing of growth, cessation of menstrual periods, hormonal disturbances, anaemia, low blood pressure and slowed heart rate. Severe cardiovascular complications can also result and in certain cases, lead to death.

If your teenager's weight drops 25% below the normal weight range for her age and height, you must talk to her doctor. She may have to be hospitalized, her treatment in this case consisting of medically-supervised realimentation. That way, her current symptoms will not get worse and she will not develop any serious new ones. Moreover, psychological treatment may be recommended to help the young woman understand how her anorexia developed and identify its causes to prevent relapse. After her stay in hospital, if indicated, this treatment can be continued on an outpatient basis.

What signs would suggest that my daughter is becoming anorexic?

Anorexia is an illness that falls in the larger category of "eating disorders". These disorders, which mainly affect teenage girls and young women, take time to heal. To help teens suffering from eating disorders, patience and parental support are required.

Here are some behaviours that could signal that your daughter is developing a problem with anorexia.

- The fear of gaining weight becomes her central preoccupation.
- She becomes literally obsessed by the fear of gaining weight, and poorly evaluates her real weight, as if when she looked in the mirror she always saw herself as fat. This suggests that she is losing her judgement about her weight, though she may brilliantly excel in other areas of her life.
- She imposes increasingly severe dietary restrictions upon herself, but denies that she is doing so. She isn't behaving in this way to annoy you but because her judgement is distorted.
- She weights herself more and more often, but denies it (again, because her judgement is distorted).
- She may make herself vomit after eating; however, not all anorexics do this.
- She may use laxatives to "purge" herself and weigh less.
- She forces herself to follow an excessive regime of physical exercise that she always finds some way of justifying.

Paradoxically, some anorexics cook a great deal. The food they prepare is meant for the other members of the family; she wants to "encourage them to eat".

It is important to mention that anorexics can occasionally or frequently be bulimic. What is bulimia? It is when a person who has been starving themselves has a sudden fit of hunger and eats a huge quantity of food in a short time, then makes themselves vomit for fear of becoming fat or from guilt.

What are the signs that our teenager is suffering from hyperactivity or an attention deficit?

The child who, before adolescence, has not been diagnosed with attention-deficit disorder, with or without hyperactivity (ADHD), probably does not display the hyperactivity component of this illness. Hyperactive children greatly disturb the people around them, so it would be unusual for a teacher, a coach or a camp counsellor not to notice and advise parents of their child's hyperactivity. Here, we will discuss attention-deficit disorder without hyperactivity.

In order to determine a case of attention-deficit, six out of the nine following symptoms must be observed over at least six months. The evaluation of this problem is unusual in that it must be based on observations made in at least two different environments, that is, at home and at school, at play and at home, etc.

Teenagers displaying attention-deficit disorder:

1) cannot pay attention to details, or make thoughtless mistakes in schoolwork and other activities;
2 have trouble sustaining their attention at school or at play;
3) do not seem to listen when someone is talking to them;
4) do not listen to instructions and cannot finish homework or domestic tasks ;

5) avoid, hate, and perform only unwillingly tasks that require sustained mental effort;
6) have difficulty planning and organizing their work and other activities;
7) often lose objects necessary for schoolwork and other activities (for example, notebooks, sports equipment, etc.);
8 become easily distracted by what is going on around them;
9) forget many things in daily life.

For several years, attention-deficit has been making the headlines due to a significant rise in the prescription of psychostimulants, such as *Ritalin®*, all over North America. An increasing number of children, and more recently teenagers and adults, are receiving this diagnosis. To this day, the exact causes of the disorder are not known. On the other hand, we know that the young people with attention deficit cannot will themselves to be calm and attentive. Research has led to theories such as heredity and brain damage. But one thing is certain: we cannot identify social factors or family tensions as being the sole cause of this disorder, though they may bring on, aggravate and prolong the problem.

Did you know?

6 to 9 boys will suffer of Attention Deficit Disorder against one girl only.

To learn more about your teen

How To Talk To Teens About Really Important Things: Specific questions and answers and useful things to say. *Charles E. Schaefer and Theresa Foy DiGeronimo.* San Francisco, Calif.: Jossey-Bass, 1999. 309 p.

How to Talk So Teens Will Listen and Listen So Teens Will Talk. *Adele Faber and Elaine Mazlish.* New York : Harper Collins, 2005. 203 p.

Parenting Teens With Love & Logic: Preparing adolescents for responsible adulthood. *Foster W. Cline and Jim Fay.* Colorado Springs, CO: Pinon Press, 2006. 317 p.

Raising Confident Boys: 100 tips for parents and teachers. *Elizabeth Hartley-Brewer.* Cambridge. Mass.: Fisher Books, 2001. 224 p. Raising Confident Girls :

100 Tips for Parents and Teachers. *Elizabeth Hartley-Brewer.* Cambridge, Mass.: Fisher Books, 2001. 224 p.

Understanding Your Teen: Parenting strategies that work. *Christine Langlois.* Mississauga, Ont.: Ballantine Books, 1999. 244 p.

Your Adolescent: Emotional, behavioral and cognitive development from early adolescence through the ten years. *David B. Pruitt.* New York: Harpers Collins, 2000. 374 p.

The Teens

Yannick Piché, on cover and page 48
Stéfany Paré, page 2
Charles-Antoine Tardif, page 8
Chloé Alchourron, page 16
Myriam Tardif, page 25
Véronique Williams, page 33
Kasmélie Doyon, page 43
Sacha C. Lemyre, page 58

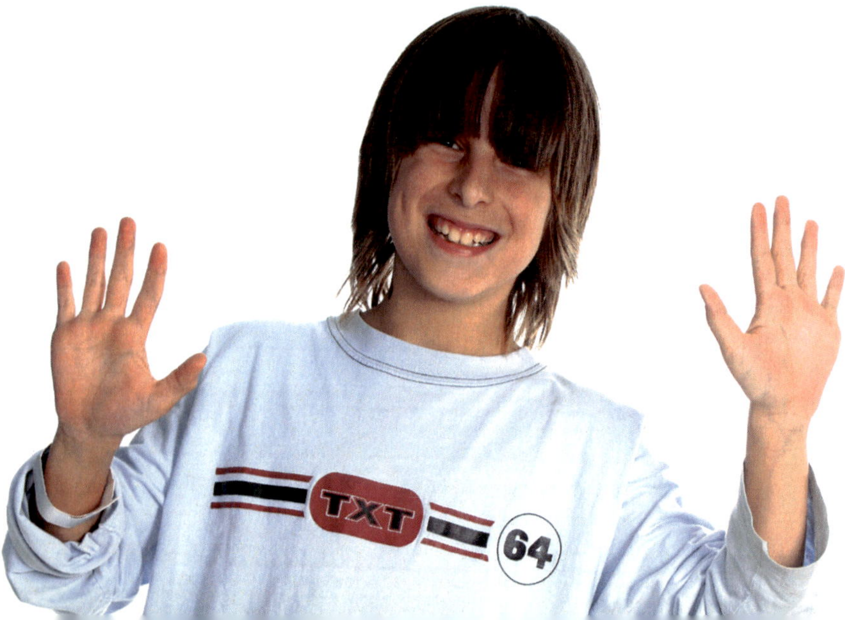

In the same collection

What Should I Know about my Child's Self-Esteem?

Germain Duclos

What Should I Know about my Child's Sexuality?

Frédérique Saint-Pierre and Marie-France Viau

What Should I Know about my Child's Development?

Francine Ferland